KETO DIET RECIPES
FOR WOMEN OVER 50

Essential Guide for Senior Women to Lose

Weight Quickly and Easily

ELIZABETH COOK

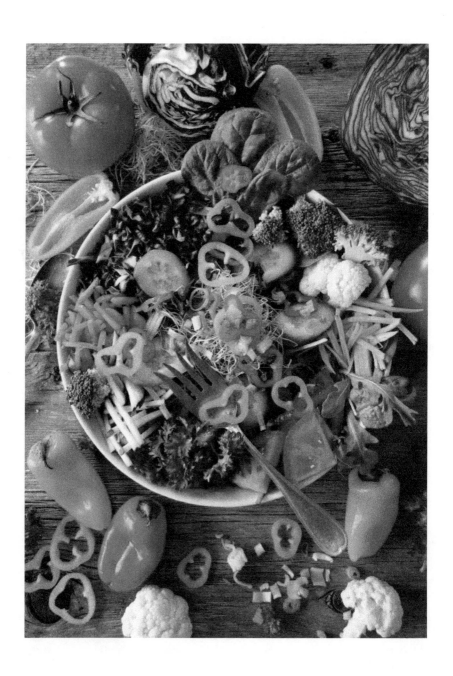

Table of Contents

Introduction

As women, when our age grows at 50, we are always looking for a quick and effective way to shed our excess weight, get our high blood sugar levels under control, reduce overall inflammation, and improve our physical and mental energy. It's frustrating to have all of these issues, especially the undeniable fats in our belly. Good thing that I found this great solution to all our worries when we reach this age level, and when our body gets weaker as time goes by. The Ketogenic diet plans.

As a woman at this age, we all know that it is much more difficult for us to lose weight than men. I have lived on a starvation level diet and exercise like a triathlete and only lose five pounds. A man will stop putting dressing on his salad and will lose twenty pounds. It just not fair. But we have the fact that we are women to blame. Women naturally have more standing between ourselves and weight loss than men do.

The mere fact that we, women, is the largest single contributor to why we find it difficult to lose weight. Since our bodies always think it needs to be prepared for a possible pregnancy, we will naturally have more body fat and less mass in our muscles than men.

Being in menopause will also cause us to add more pounds to our bodies, especially in the lower half. After menopause, our metabolism naturally slows down. Our hormones levels will decrease. These two factors alone will cause weight gain in the post-menopausal period.

There are numerous diet plan options offered to help shed weight, but the Ketogenic diet has been the most preferred lately. We've got many concerns around keto's effectiveness and exactly how to follow the diet plan in a healthy and balanced means.

The ketogenic diet for ladies at the age or over 50 is an easy and ideal way to shed extra pounds, stay energetic, and enjoy a healthy life. It does not only balances hormones but also improves our body capabilities without causing any harm to our overall wellness. Thus, if you are fighting with post-menopausal symptoms and other health issues, you should do a Keto diet right away!

A Keto diet is a lifestyle, not a diet so, treat it like the same. The best way to approach keto to gain maximum benefits, especially for women over 50s, is to treat it as a lifestyle. You can't restrict your meal intake through obstructive and strict diets forever, right? It's the fundamental reason fad diets fail — we limit ourselves from too much to get rapid results, then we're are right back again at the weight where we started, or God forbid worse.

Keto is not a kind of diet that can be followed strictly forever — unless you need it as a therapeutic diet (i.e., epilepsy), a very narrow category. In keto diet, we slowly transit into a curative state that we can withstand forever in a healthier way.

So, for me, being on a keto diet does not mean that I will be in ketosis forever. Instead, it means letting myself love consideration, such as a few desserts while vacationing or partying. It does not set me back to enjoy these desserts and let me consider it as the end of the diet. I can wake up the following morning and go back to the keto lifestyle, most suitable for me and my body consistently.

It allows my body to boost its fat loss drastically in many cases, which helps in decreasing pockets of undesirable fat.

With Keto Diet, it's not only giving weight loss assistance to reduce my weight, yet it can likewise ward off yearnings for unhealthy foods and protect me against calories collisions throughout the day. That is why I want it to share with you how promising this Keto diet. As our age grow older, we must not let our body do the same. Focus your mindset on this fantastic diet, read, apply, and enjoy its best benefits.

Breakfast Recipes

1.   Cheese Crepes

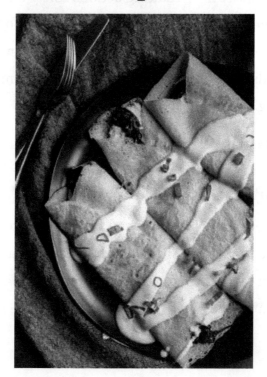

Preparation time: 15 minutes

Cooking time: 20 minutes

Servings: 5

Ingredients:

- 6 ounces cream cheese

- 1/3 cup Parmesan cheese

- 6 large organic eggs

- 1 teaspoon granulated erythritol

- 1 1/2 tablespoon coconut flour

- 1/8 teaspoon xanthan gum

- 2 tablespoons unsalted butter

Directions:

1. Pulse the cream cheese, Parmesan cheese, eggs, and erythritol using a blender.

2. Place the coconut flour and xanthan gum and pulse again.

3. Now, pulse on medium speed. Transfer and put aside within 5 minutes.

4. Melt butter over medium-low heat.

5. Place 1 portion of the mixture and tilt the pan to spread into a thin layer.

6. Cook within 1½ minutes.

7. Flip the crepe and cook within 15-20 seconds more. Serve.

Nutrition:

Calories 297

Net Carbs 1.9 g

Total Fat 25.1 g

Cholesterol 281 mg

Total Carbs 3.5 g

Protein 13.7 g

2.   Ricotta Pancakes

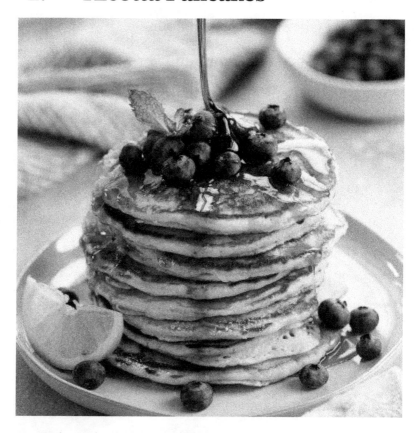

Preparation time: 10 minutes

Cooking time: 20 minutes

Servings: 4

Ingredients:

- 4 organic eggs

- ½ cup ricotta cheese

- ¼ cup vanilla whey protein powder

- ½ teaspoon organic baking powder

- salt

- ½ teaspoon liquid stevia

- 2 tablespoons unsalted butter

Directions:

1. Pulse all the fixing in the blender. Warm-up butter over medium heat. Put the batter and spread it evenly.

2. Cook within 2 minutes. Flip and cook again within 1–2 minutes. Serve.

Nutrition:

Calories 184

Net Carbs 2.7 g

Total Fat 12.9 g

Total Carbs 2.7 g

Sugar 0.8 g

Protein 14.6 g

3. Yogurt Waffles

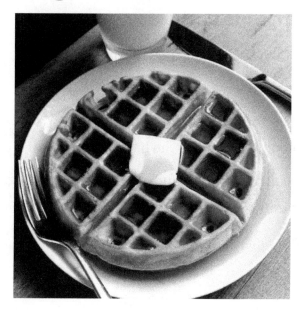

Preparation time: 15 minutes

Cooking time: 25 minutes

Servings: 5

Ingredients:

- ½ cup golden flax seeds meal
- ½ cup plus 3 tablespoons almond flour
- 1-1½ tablespoons granulated erythritol
- 1 tablespoon vanilla whey protein powder
- ¼ teaspoon baking soda
- ½ teaspoon organic baking powder
- ¼ teaspoon xanthan gum

- Salt

- 1 large organic egg

- 1 organic egg

- 2 tablespoons unsweetened almond milk

- 1½ tablespoons unsalted butter

- 3 ounces plain Greek yogurt

Directions:

1. Preheat the waffle iron and then grease it.

2. Mix add the flour, erythritol, protein powder, baking soda, baking powder, xanthan gum, and salt.

3. Beat the egg white until stiff peaks. In a third bowl, add 2 egg yolks, whole egg, almond milk, butter, and yogurt, and beat.

4. Put egg mixture into the bowl of the flour mixture and mix.

5. Gently, fold in the beaten egg whites. Place ¼ cup of the mixture into preheated waffle iron and cook for about 4–5 minutes. Serve.

Nutrition:

Calories 250

Net Carbs 3.2 g

Total Fat 18.7 g

Protein 8.4 g

4.   Broccoli Muffins

Preparation time: 15 minutes

Cooking time: 20 minutes

Servings: 6

Ingredients:

- 2 tablespoons unsalted butter
- 6 large organic eggs
- ½ cup heavy whipping cream
- ½ cup Parmesan cheese
- Salt & ground black pepper
- 1¼ cups broccoli
- 2 tablespoons parsley
- ½ cup Swiss cheese

Directions:

1. Warm-up oven to 350°F, then grease a 12-cup muffin tin.

2. Mix the eggs, cream, Parmesan cheese, salt, and black pepper.

3. Divide the broccoli and parsley in the muffin cup.

4. Top with the egg mixture, with Swiss cheese.

5. Bake within 20 minutes. Cool for about 5 minutes. Serve.

Nutrition:

Calories 231

Net Carbs 2 g

Total Fat 18.1 g

Cholesterol 228 mg

Sodium 352 mg

Protein 13.5 g

5. Pumpkin Bread

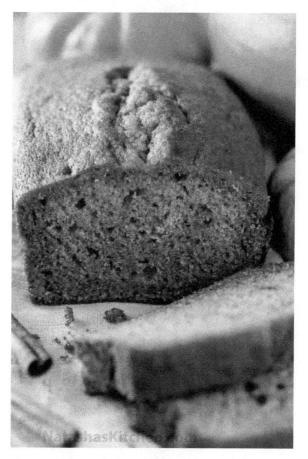

Preparation time: 15 minutes

Cooking time: 1 hour

Servings: 16

Ingredients:

- 1 2/3 cups almond flour
- 1½ teaspoons organic baking powder
- ½ teaspoon pumpkin pie spice

- ½ teaspoon cinnamon

- ½ teaspoon cloves

- ½ teaspoon salt

- 8 ounces cream cheese

- 6 organic eggs

- 1 tablespoon coconut flour

- 1 cup powdered erythritol

- 1 teaspoon stevia powder

- 1 teaspoon organic lemon extract

- 1 cup pumpkin puree

- ½ cup of coconut oil

Directions:

1. Warm-up oven to 325°F. Grease 2 bread loaf pans.

2. Mix almond flour, baking powder, spices, and salt in a small bowl.

3. In a second bowl, add the cream cheese, 1 egg, coconut flour, ¼ cup of erythritol, and ¼ teaspoon of the stevia, and beat.

4. In a third bowl, add the pumpkin puree, oil, 5 eggs, ¾ cup of the erythritol, and ¾ teaspoon of the stevia and mix.

5. Mix the pumpkin mixture into the bowl of the flour mixture.

6. Place about ¼ of the pumpkin mixture into each loaf pan.

7. Top each pan with the cream cheese mixture, plus the rest pumpkin mixture.

8. Bake within 50–60 minutes. Cold within 10 minutes. Slice and serve.

Nutrition:

Calories 216

Net Carbs 2.5 g

Total Fat 19.8 g

Cholesterol 77 mg

Sodium 140 mg

Protein 3.4 g

6.   Eggs in Avocado Cups

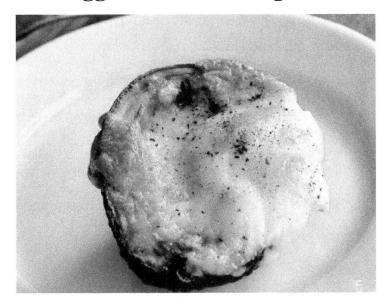

Preparation time: 10 minutes

Cooking time: 20 minutes

Servings: 4

Ingredients:

- 2 avocados
- 4 organic eggs
- Salt
- Ground black pepper
- 4 tablespoons cheddar cheese
- 2 cooked bacon
- 1 tablespoon scallion greens

Directions:

1. Warm-up oven to 400°F. Remove 2 tablespoons of flesh from the avocado.

2. Place avocado halves into a small baking dish.

3. Crack an egg in each avocado half and sprinkle with salt plus black pepper.

4. Top each egg with cheddar cheese evenly.

5. Bake within 20 minutes. Serve with bacon and chives.

Nutrition:

Calories 343

Net Carbs 2.2 g

Total Fat 29.1 g

Cholesterol 186 mg

Sodium 372 mg

Protein 13.8 g

7.　Cheddar Scramble

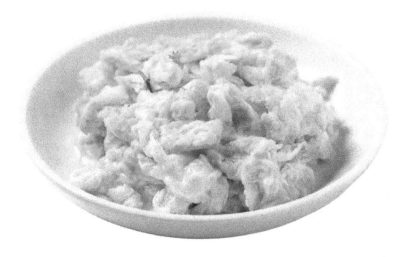

Preparation time: 10 minutes

Cooking time: 8 minutes

Servings: 6

Ingredients:

- 2 tablespoons olive oil

- 1 small yellow onion

- 12 large organic eggs

- Salt and ground black pepper

- 4 ounces cheddar cheese

Directions;

1. Warm-up oil over medium heat.

2. Sauté the onion within 4–5 minutes.

3. Add the eggs, salt, and black pepper and cook within 3 minutes.

4. Remove then stir in the cheese. Serve.

Nutrition:

Calories 264

Net Carbs 1.8 g

Total Fat 20.9 g

Cholesterol 392 mg

Sodium 285 mg

Protein 17.4 g

8.   Bacon Omelet

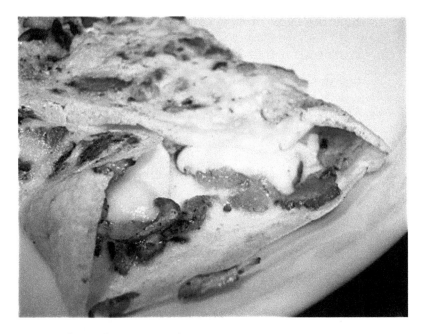

Preparation time: 10 minutes

Cooking time: 15 minutes

Servings: 2

Ingredients:

- 4 organic eggs
- 1 tablespoon chives
- Salt
- ground black pepper
- 4 bacon slices
- 1 tablespoon unsalted butter
- 2 ounces cheddar cheese

Directions:

1. Beat the eggs, chives, salt, and black pepper in a bowl.

2. Warm-up a pan over medium-high heat then cooks the bacon slices within 8–10 minutes.

3. Chop the bacon slices. Melt butter and cook the egg mixture within 2 minutes.

4. Flip the omelet and top with chopped bacon. Cook within 1–2 minutes.

5. Remove then put the cheese in the center of the omelet. Serve.

Nutrition:

Calories 427

Net Carbs 1.2 g

Total Fat 28.2 g

Cholesterol 469 mg

Sodium 668 mg

Sugar 1 g

Protein 29.1 g

9.   Green Veggies Quiche

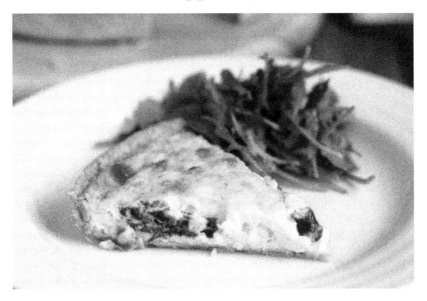

Preparation time: 20 minutes

Cooking time: 20 minutes

Servings: 4

Ingredients:

- 6 organic eggs
- ½ cup unsweetened almond milk
- Salt and ground black pepper
- 2 cups baby spinach
- ½ cup green bell pepper
- 1 scallion
- ¼ cup cilantro
- 1 tablespoon chives,

- 3 tablespoons mozzarella cheese

Directions:

1. Warm-up oven to 400°F.

2. Grease a pie dish. Beat eggs, almond milk, salt, and black pepper. Set aside.

3. In another bowl, add the vegetables and herbs then mix.

4. Place the veggie mixture and top with the egg mixture in the pie dish.

5. Bake within 20 minutes. Remove then sprinkle with the Parmesan cheese.

6. Slice and serve.

Nutrition:

Calories 176

Net Carbs 4.1 g

Total Fat 10.9 g

Cholesterol 257 mg

Sugar 4 g

Protein 15.4 g

10. Chicken & Asparagus Frittata

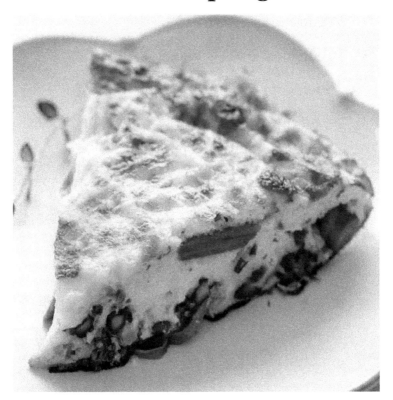

Preparation time: 15 minutes

Cooking time: 12 minutes

Servings: 4

Ingredients:

- ½ cup grass-fed chicken breast
- 1/3 cup Parmesan cheese
- 6 organic eggs
- Salt
- ground black pepper

- 1/3 cup boiled asparagus

- ¼ cup cherry tomatoes

- ¼ cup mozzarella cheese

Directions:

1. Warm-up broiler of the oven, then mix Parmesan cheese, eggs, salt, and black pepper in a bowl.

2. Melt butter, then cooks the chicken and asparagus within 2–3 minutes.

3. Add the egg mixture and tomatoes and mix. Cook within 4–5 minutes.

4. Remove then sprinkle with the Parmesan cheese.

5. Transfer the wok under the broiler and broil within 3–4 minutes. Slice and serve.

Nutrition:

Calories 158

Net Carbs 1.3 g

Total Fat 9.3 g

Cholesterol 265 mg

Sodium 267 mg

Sugar 1 g

Lunch Recipes

11. Easy Keto Smoked Salmon Lunch Bowl.

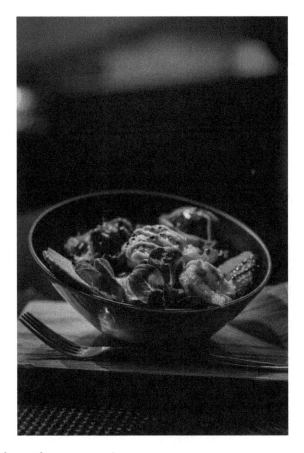

Preparation time: 15 minutes

Cooking time: 0 minutes

Servings: 2

Ingredients:

- Twelve-ounce smoked salmon
- 4 tablespoon mayonnaise
- Two-ounce spinach
- One tablespoon olive oil
- One medium lime
- Pepper
- Salt

Directions:

1. Arrange the mayonnaise, salmon, spinach on a plate. Sprinkle olive oil over the spinach.

2. Serve with lime wedges and put salt plus pepper.

Nutrition:

457 calories

1.9g net carbs

34.8g fats

32.3g protein.

12.   Easy One-Pan Ground Beef and Green Beans

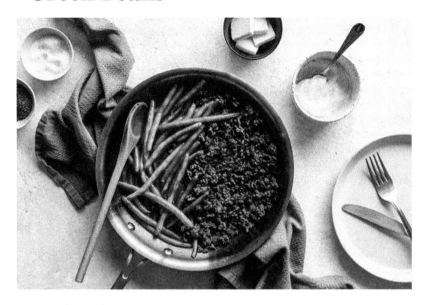

Preparation time: 15 minutes

Cooking time: 15 minutes

Servings: 2

Ingredients:

- Ten ounces ground beef

- Nine ounces green beans

- Pepper

- salt

- Two tablespoons sour cream

- 3½ ounces butter

Directions:

1. Warm-up the butter to a pan over high heat.

2. Put the ground beef plus the pepper and salt. Cook.

3. Reduce heat to medium. Add the remaining butter and the green beans then cook within five minutes. Put pepper and salt, then transfer. Serve with a dollop of sour cream.

Nutrition:

6.65g Net Carbs

787.5 Calories

71.75g Fats

27.5g Protein.

13. Easy Spinach and Bacon Salad

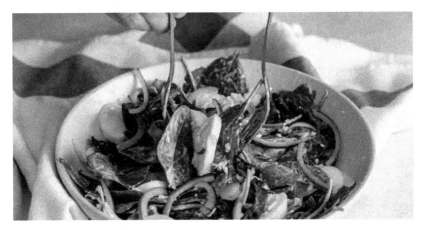

Preparation time: 15 minutes

Cooking time: 15 minutes

Servings: 4

Ingredients:

- Eight ounces spinach

- Four large hard-boiled eggs

- 6 ounces bacon

- Two medium red onion

- Two cup mayonnaise

- Pepper

- salt

Directions:

1. Cook the bacon, then chop into pieces, set aside.

2. Slice the hard-boiled eggs, and then rinse the spinach.

3. Combine the lettuce, mayonnaise, and bacon fat into a large cup, put pepper and salt.

4. Add the red onion, sliced eggs, and bacon into the salad, then toss. Serve.

Nutrition:

45.9g Fats

509.15 Calories

2.5g Net Carbs

19.75g protein

14. Easy Keto Italian Plate

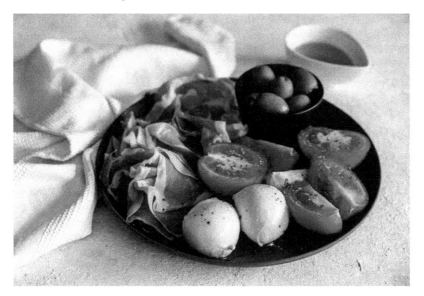

Preparation time: 15 minutes

Cooking time: 0 minutes

Servings: 2

Ingredients:

- Seven ounces mozzarella cheese

- Seven ounces prosciutto

- Two tomatoes

- Four tablespoons olive oil

- Ten whole green olives

- Pepper

- salt

Directions:

1. Arrange the tomato, olives, mozzarella, and prosciutto on a plate.

2. Season the tomato and cheese with pepper and salt. Serve with olive oil.

Nutrition:

780.98 Calories

5.9g Net Carbs

60.74g Fats

50.87g protein.

15.   Fresh Broccoli and Dill Keto Salad

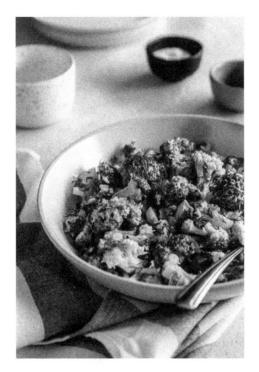

Preparation time: 15 minutes

Cooking time: 7 minutes

Servings: 3

Ingredients:

- 16 ounces broccoli

- One/Two cup mayonnaise

- 3/4 cup chopped dill

- Salt

- pepper

Directions:

1. Boil salted water in a saucepan. Put the chopped broccoli to the pot and boil for 3-5 minutes. Drain and set aside. Once cooled, mix the rest of the fixing. Put pepper and salt, then serve.

Nutrition:

303.33 Calories

6.2g Net Carbs

28.1g Fats

4.03g Protein.

16. Keto Smoked Salmon Filled Avocados.

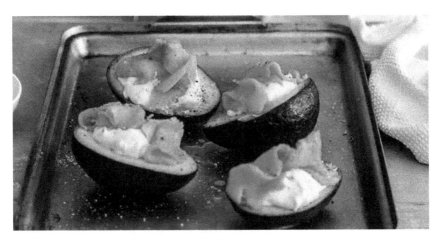

Preparation time: 15 minutes

Cooking time: 0 minutes

Servings: 1

Ingredients:

- One avocado
- Three ounces smoked salmon
- Four tablespoons sour cream
- One tablespoon lemon juice
- Pepper
- salt

Directions:

1. Cut the avocado into two. Place the sour cream in the hollow parts of the avocado with smoked salmon. Put pepper and salt, squeeze lemon juice over the top. Serve.

Nutrition:

517 Calories

6.7g Net Carbs

42.6g Fats

20.6g Protein

17. Low-Carb Broccoli Lemon Parmesan Soup

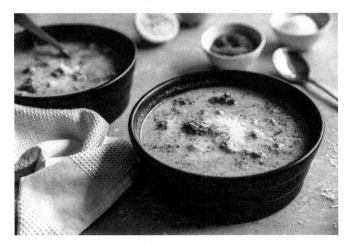

Preparation time: 15 minutes

Cooking time: 15 minutes

Servings: 4

Ingredients:

- Three cups of water

- One cup unsweetened almond milk

- Thirty-two ounces broccoli florets

- One cup heavy whipping cream

- 3/4 cup Parmesan cheese

- Salt

- pepper

- Two tablespoons lemon juice

Directions:

1. Cook broccoli plus water over medium-high heat.

2. Take out 1 cup of the cooking liquid, and remove the rest.

3. Blend half the broccoli, reserved cooking oil, unsweetened almond milk, heavy cream, and salt plus pepper in a blender.

4. Put the blended items to the remaining broccoli, and stir with Parmesan cheese and lemon juice. Cook until heated through. Serve with Parmesan cheese on the top.

Nutrition:

371 Calories

11.67g Net Carbs

28.38g Fats

14.63g Protein

18. Prosciutto and Mozzarella Bomb

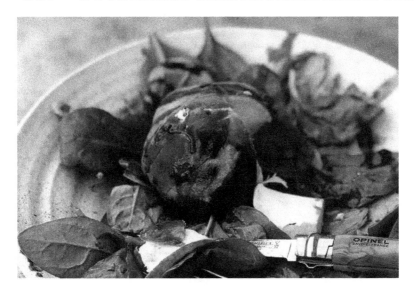

Preparation time: 15 minutes

Cooking time: 10 minutes

Servings: 4

Ingredients:

- Four ounces sliced prosciutto

- Eight ounces mozzarella ball

- Olive oil

Directions:

1. Layer half of the prosciutto vertically. Lay the remaining slices horizontally across the first set of slices. Place mozzarella ball, upside down, onto the crisscrossed prosciutto slices.

2. Wrap the mozzarella ball with the prosciutto slices. Warm-up the olive oil in a skillet, crisp the prosciutto, then serve.

Nutrition:

253 Calories

1.08g Net Carbs

19.35g Fats

18g Protein

19. Summer Tuna Avocado Salad

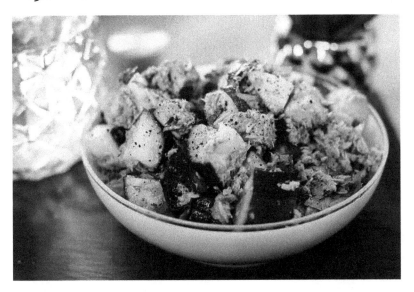

Preparation time: 15 minutes

Cooking time: 0 minutes

Servings: 2

Ingredients:

- 1can tuna flake

- One medium avocado

- One medium English cucumber

- ¼ cup cilantro

- One tablespoon lemon juice

- One tablespoon olive oil

- Pepper

- salt

Directions:

1. Put the first 4 ingredients into a salad bowl. Sprinkle with the lemon and olive oil. Serve.

Nutrition:

303 Calories

5.2g Net Carbs

22.6g Fats

16.7g Protein.

20. Mushrooms & Goat Cheese Salad

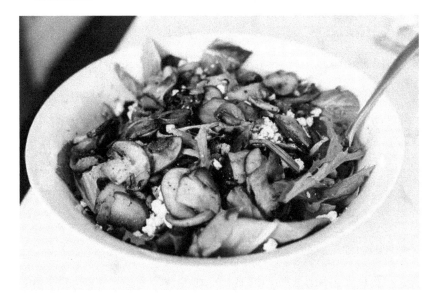

Preparation time: 15 minutes

Cooking time: 10 minutes

Servings: 1

Ingredients:

- One tablespoon butter
- Two ounces cremini mushrooms
- Pepper
- salt
- Four ounces spring mix
- One-ounce cooked bacon
- One-ounce goat cheese

- One tablespoon olive oil

- One tablespoon balsamic vinegar

Directions:

1. Sautee the mushrooms, put pepper and salt.

2. Place the salad greens in a bowl. Top with goat cheese and crumbled bacon.

3. Mix these in the salad once the mushrooms are done.

4. Whisk the olive oil in a small bowl and balsamic vinegar. Put the salad on top and serve.

Nutrition:

243 Cal 21 gram total fat 8 gram carb

4 gram saturated fat1 gram fiber

Snacks and Cakes

21. Keto Raspberry Cake and White Chocolate Sauce

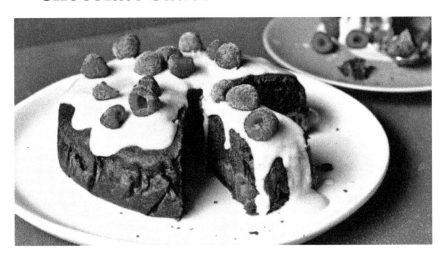

Preparation Time: 15 minutes

Cooking Time: 45 minutes

Servings: 4

Ingredients:

- 5 ounces cacao butter

- 4 teaspoons pure vanilla extract

- 4 eggs

- 3 cup raspberries

- 2½ ounces grass-fed ghee

- 1 teaspoon baking powder

- 1 tablespoon apple cider vinegar

- 1 cup green banana flour

- ¾ cup coconut cream

- ¾ cup granulated sweetener

- 4 ounces cacao butter

- 2 teaspoons pure vanilla extract

- ¾ cup coconut cream

- salt

Directions:

1. Mix the butter and the sweetener. Pour in the grass-fed ghee into the mix, blend.

2. Beat the eggs in a different bowl.

3. Warm-up oven to 350 degrees F. Grease a baking pan.

4. Put the mixed eggs to the butter and sweetener mixture. Mix well.

5. Pour in the banana flour and mix. Then the vanilla extract, apple cider, coconut cream, baking powder, and mix again.

6. Spoon around the sliced raspberries. Then, sprinkle flour in the baking pan.

7. Put the mixture into the pan then bake within 45 minutes. Cool down.

8. For the sauce

9. Mix cacao butter with 2 teaspoons pure vanilla extract. Add coconut cream and beat. Put salt and beat. Chop the remaining berries and throw them in the mix. Pour the mix on the cake. Serve cold.

Nutrition:

Calories: 325 kcal

Total Fat: 12g

Total Carbs: 3g

Protein: 40g

22. Keto Chocolate Chip Cookies

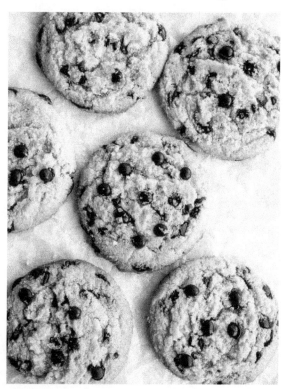

Preparation Time: 15 minutes

Cooking Time: 10 minutes

Servings: 4

Ingredients:

- 7 spoons unsweetened coconut powder
- 7 tablespoons Keto chocolate chips
- 5 tablespoons butter
- 2 flat tablespoon baking powder
- 2 eggs

- 2/3 confectioners swerve

- 1 1/3 cups almond flour

- A teaspoon vanilla extract

Directions

1. Warm-up oven to 325.

2. Melt half chocolate chips, then the butter. Mix.

3. Mix the eggs in chocolate and butter mixture.

4. Mix in the vanilla extract, coconut powder, confectioners swerve, and almond flour. Mix well.

5. Add chocolate chip cookies. Then, add baking powder, and mix until dough forms.

6. Spread out and cut out cookies, top with chocolate chips.

7. Bake within 8 to 10 minutes. Serve.

Nutrition:

Calories: 287 kcal

Total Fat: 19g

Total Carbs: 6.5g

Protein: 6.8g

23. Keto Beef and Sausage Balls

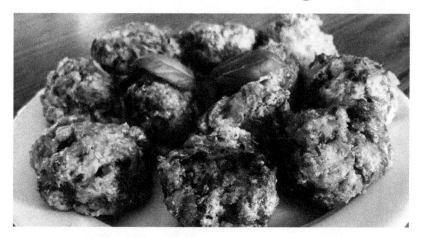

Preparation Time: 15 minutes

Cooking Time: 20 minutes

Servings: 3

Ingredients:

- Meat

- 2 pounds ground beef

- 2 pounds ground sausage

- 2 eggs

- ½ cup Keto mayonnaise

- 1/3 cup ground pork rinds

- ½ cup Parmesan cheese

- Salt

- Pepper

- 2 tablespoons butter

- 3 tablespoons oil

Sauce

- 3 diced onions

- 2 pounds mushrooms

- 5 cloves garlic

- 3 cups beef broth

- 1 cup sour cream

- 2 tablespoons mustard

- Worcestershire sauce

- Salt

- Pepper

- Parsley

- 1 tablespoon Arrowroot powder

Directions:

1. Put meat, egg, and onions in a bowl, mix. Put beef, parmesan, egg, mayonnaise, sausage, pork rind in a bowl. Add salt and pepper. Warm-up oil in a skillet.

2. Mold the beef mixture into balls, fry within 7-10 minutes. Put aside.

3. Fry the diced onions, then the garlic and mushrooms, cook within 3 minutes. Then, add the broth.

4. Mix in mustard, sour cream, and Worcestershire sauce. Boil within two minutes, then adds in the meatballs. Add salt and pepper, simmer. Serve.

Nutrition:

Calories: 592 kcal

Total Fat: 53.9g

Total Carbs: 1.3g

Protein: 25.4g

24. Keto Coconut Flake Balls

Preparation Time: 15 minutes

Cooking Time: 0 minutes

Servings: 2

Ingredients:

- 1 Vanilla Shortbread Collagen Protein Bar

- 1 tablespoon lemon

- ¼ teaspoon ground ginger

- ½ cup unsweetened coconut flakes,

- ¼ teaspoon ground turmeric

Directions:

1. Process protein bar, ginger, turmeric, and ¾ of the total bits into a food processor.

2. Remove and add a spoon of water and roll till dough forms.

3. Roll into balls, and sprinkle the rest of the flakes on it. Serve.

Nutrition:

Calories: 204 kcal

Total Fat: 11g

Total Carbs: 4.2g

Protein: 1.5g

25.   Keto Chocolate Greek Yoghurt Cookies

Preparation Time: 15 minutes

Cooking Time: 30 minutes

Servings: 3

Ingredients:

- 3 eggs

- 1/8 teaspoon tartar

- 5 tablespoons softened Greek yogurt

Directions:

1. Beat the egg whites, the tartar, and mix.

2. In the yolk, put in the Greek yogurt, and mix.

3. Combine both egg whites and yolk batter into a bowl.

4. Bake within 25-30 minutes, serve.

Nutrition:

Calories: 287 kcal

Total Fat: 19g

Total Carbs: 6.5g

Protein: 6.8g

26.   Keto coconut flavored ice cream

Preparation Time: 15 minutes

Cooking Time: 0 minutes

Servings: 4

Ingredients:

4 cups of coconut milk

2/3 cup xylitol

¼ teaspoon salt

2 teaspoons vanilla extract

1 teaspoon coconut extract

Directions:

Add the coconut milk in a bowl, with the sweetener, extracts, and salt. Mix.

Pour this mixture in the ice cube trays, and put it in the freezer. Serve.

Nutrition:

Calories: 244 kcal

Total Fat: 48g

Total Carbs: 6g

Protein: 15g

27.   Chocolate-Coconut Cookies

Preparation Time: 15 minutes

Cooking Time: 20 minutes

Servings: 4

Ingredients:

- 2 eggs

- ½ cup of cocoa powder

- ½ cup flour

- ½ cup of coconut oil

- ¼ cup grated coconut

- Stevia

Directions:

1. Warm-up oven to 350 °F. Crack eggs and separate whites and yolks, mix separately.

2. Put salt to the yolks. Warm-up oil in a skillet, and add cocoa, egg whites, mixing, add in the salted yolks. Then, add stevia. Add in coconut flour, and mix until dough forms.

3. On a flat surface, sprinkle grated coconut. Roll the dough around in the coconut, mix. Mold into cookies. Bake within 15 minutes, serve.

Nutrition:

Calories: 260 kcal

Total Fat: 26g

Total Carbs: 4.5g

Protein: 1g

28. Keto Buffalo Chicken Meatballs

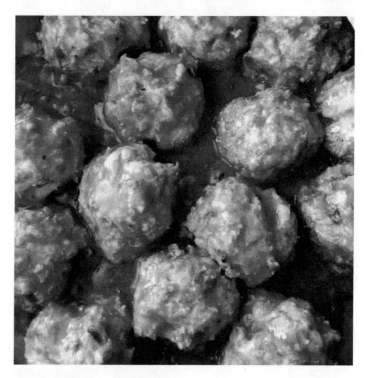

Preparation Time: 15 minutes

Cooking Time: 20 minutes

Servings: 3

Ingredients:

- 1-pound ground chicken

- 1 large

- 2/3 cup hot sauce

- ½ cup almond flour

- ½ teaspoon salt

- ½ teaspoon pepper

- ½ cup melted butter

- 1 large onion

- 1 teaspoon garlic

Directions:

1. Combine meat, egg, and onions in a bowl. Pour in almond flour, garlic, salt, and pepper in.

2. Warm-up oven to 350°F and grease a baking tray.

3. Mold the egg mixture into balls. Bake within 18-20 minutes.

4. Melt butter in the microwave for few seconds; mix it with hot sauce.

5. Put the sauce into meatballs. Serve.

Nutrition:

Calories: 360 kcal

Total Fat: 26g

Total Carbs: 4.5g

Protein: 1g

29. Eggplant And Chickpea Bites

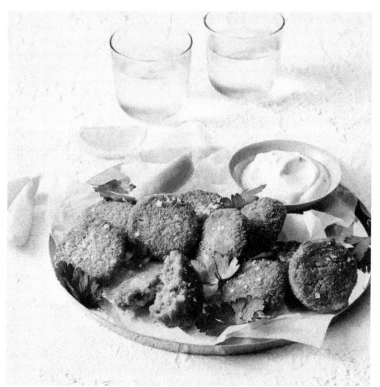

Preparation Time: 15 minutes

Cooking Time: 90 minutes

Servings: 6

Ingredients:

- 3 large aubergines

- Spray oil

- 2 large cloves garlic

- 2 tablespoon. coriander powder

- 2 tablespoon. cumin seeds

- 400 g canned chickpeas

- 2 Tablespoon. chickpea flour

- Zest and juice 1/2 lemon

- 1/2 lemon quartered

- 3 tablespoon. tablespoon polenta

Directions:

1. Warm-up oven to 200°C. Grease the eggplant halves and place it on the meat side up on a baking sheet.

2. Sprinkle with coriander and cumin seeds, and then place the cloves of garlic on the plate. Roast within 40 minutes, put aside.

3. Add chickpeas, chickpea flour, zest, and lemon juice. Crush roughly and mix well.

4. Form about twenty pellets and place them on a baking sheet. Fridge within 30 minutes.

5. Warm-up oven to 180°C. Remove the meatballs from the fridge and coat it in the polenta. Roast for 20 minutes. Serve with lemon wedges.

Nutrition:

Calories: 70

Carbs: 4g

Fat: 5g

Protein: 2g

30. Baba Ganoush

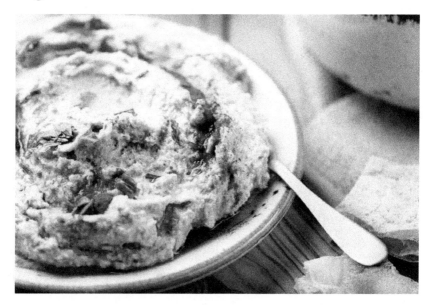

Preparation Time: 15 minutes

Cooking Time: 20 minutes

Servings: 3

Ingredients:

- 1 large aubergine
- 1 head of garlic
- 30 ml of olive oil
- Lemon juice

Directions:

1. Warm-up oven to 350 ° F.
2. Place the eggplant on the plate, skin side up. Roast, about 1 hour.

3. Place the garlic cloves in a square of aluminum foil. Fold the edges of the sheet. Roast with the eggplant, about 20 minutes. Let cool. Purée the pods with a garlic press.

4. Puree the flesh of the eggplant. Add the garlic puree, the oil, and the lemon juice.

5. Serve.

Nutrition:

Calories: 87

Carbs: 6g

Fat: 6g

Protein: 2g

Dinner

31.   Baked Fish Fillets with Vegetables in Foil

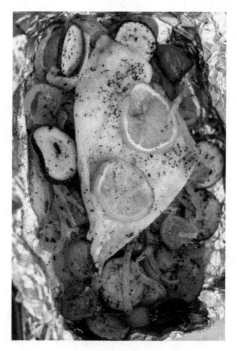

Preparation time: 15 minutes

Cooking time: 40 minutes

Servings: 3

Ingredients:

- 1 lb. cod

- 1 red bell pepper

- 6 cherry tomatoes

- 1 leek
- ¼ onion
- ½ zucchini
- 1 clove garlic
- 2 tablespoon olives
- 1 oz butter
- 2 tablespoon olive oil
- ½ lemon sliced
- Coriander leaves
- Salt
- pepper

Directions:

1. Warm-up oven to 400°F. Transfer all the vegetables to a baking sheet lined with foil.
2. Cut the fish into bite-sized and add to the vegetables. Add salt and pepper, olive oil and add pieces of butter. Bake for 35 – 40 minutes. Serve.

Nutrition:

Calories 339

Fat 19g

Protein 35g

Carbs 5g

32.   Fish & Chips

Preparation time: 15 minutes

Cooking time: 30 minutes

Servings: 2

Ingredients:

For chips:

- ½ tablespoon olive oil

- 1 medium zucchini

- Salt

- pepper

- For fish:

- ¾ lb. cod

- Oil

- ½ cup almond flour

- ¼ teaspoon onion powder

For Sauce:

- 2 tablespoon dill pickle relish

- ¼ tablespoon curry powder

- ½ cup mayonnaise

- ½ teaspoon paprika powder

- ½ cup parmesan cheese

- 1 egg

- Salt

- pepper

Directions:

1. Mix all the sauce fixing in a bowl. Set aside.

2. Warm-up oven to 400°F. Make thin zucchini rods, brush with oil, and spread on the baking sheet. Put salt and pepper then bake within 30 minutes.

3. Beat the egg in a bowl. On a separate plate, combine the parmesan cheese, almond flour, and the remaining spices.

4. Slice the fish into 1 inch by 1-inch pieces. Roll them on the flour mixture. Dip in the beaten egg and then in the flour again. Fry the fish for three minutes. Serve.

Nutrition:

Calories 463

Fat 26.2 g

Protein 49g

Carbs 6g

33. Baked Salmon with Almonds and Cream Sauce

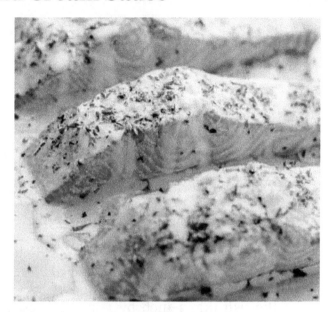

Preparation time: 10 minutes

Cooking time: 20 minutes

Servings: 2

Ingredients:

Almond Crumbs Creamy Sauce

3 tablespoon almonds

2 tablespoon almond milk

½ cup cream cheese

Salt

Fish

1 salmon fillet

1 teaspoon coconut oil

1 tablespoon lemon zest

1 teaspoon salt

White pepper

Directions:

Cut the salmon in half. Rub the salmon with the lemon zest, salt and pepper. Marinade for 20 minutes.

Fry the fish on both sides. Top with almond crumbs and bake within 10 to 15 minutes.

Remove and put aside.

Place the baking dish on fire and add the cream cheese. Combine the fish baking juices and the cheese. Mix, then pour the sauce onto the fish. Serve.

Nutrition:

Calories 522

Fat 44g

Protein 28g

Carbs 2.4g

34. Shrimp and Sausage Bake

Preparation time: 15 minutes

Cooking time: 20 minutes

Servings: 4

Ingredients:

- 2 tablespoon olive oil
- 6 ounces chorizo sausage
- ½ pound shrimp
- ½ small sweet onion
- 1 teaspoon garlic
- ¼ cup Herbed Chicken Stock
- Pinch red pepper flakes
- 1 red bell pepper

Directions:

1. Sauté the sausage within 6 minutes. Add the shrimp and sauté within 4 minutes. Remove both and set aside.

2. Cook the red pepper, onion, and garlic to the skillet within 4 minutes. Put the chicken stock along with the cooked sausage and shrimp. Simmer for 3 minutes.

3. Stir in the red pepper flake and serve.

Nutrition:

Calories 323

Fat 24g

Protein 20g

Carbs 6g

35. Herb Butter Scallops

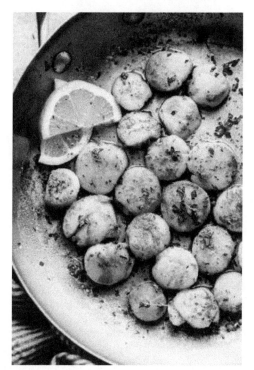

Preparation time: 10 minutes

Cooking time: 10 minutes

Servings: 4

Ingredients:

- 1-pound sea scallops

- ground black pepper

- 8 tablespoon butter

- 2 teaspoon garlic

- 1 lemon juice

- 2 teaspoon basil

- 1 teaspoon thyme

Directions:

1. Pat dry the scallops then put pepper. Sear each side within 2 ½ minutes per side.

2. Remove then set aside. Sauté the garlic within 3 minutes. Stir in the lemon juice, basil and thyme and return the scallops to the skillet, mix.

3. Serve.

Nutrition:

Calories 306

Fat 24g

Protein 19g

Carbs 4g

36. Pan-Seared Halibut with Citrus Butter Sauce

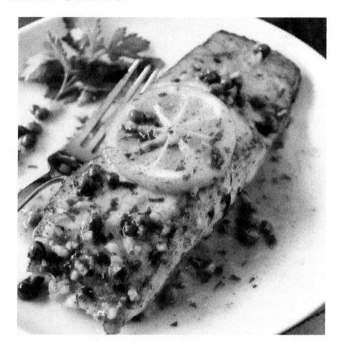

Preparation time: 10 minutes

Cooking time: 15 minutes

Servings: 4

Ingredients:

- 4 halibut fillets

- Sea salt

- ground pepper

- ¼ cup butter

- 2 tablespoon garlic

- 1 shallot

- 3 tablespoons dry white wine

- 1 tablespoon orange juice

- 1 tablespoon lemon juice

- 2 teaspoon parsley

- 2 teaspoon olive oil

Directions:

1. Pat dry the fish then put salt and pepper. Set aside.

2. Sauté the garlic and shallot within 3 minutes.

3. Whisk in the white wine, lemon juice, and orange juice and simmer within 2 minutes.

4. Remove the sauce and stir in the parsley; set aside.

5. Panfry the fish until within 10 minutes. Serve with sauce.

Nutrition:

Calories 319

Fat 26g

Protein 22g

Carbs 2g

37.   Baked Coconut Haddock

Preparation time: 10 minutes

Cooking time: 12 minutes

Servings: 4

Ingredients:

- 4 (5 oz) boneless haddock fillets
- Sea salt
- Freshly ground pepper
- 1 cup shredded unsweetened coconut
- ½ cup ground hazelnuts
- 2 tablespoon coconut oil, melted

Directions:

1. Warm oven to 400°F.

2. Pat dry fillets and lightly season them with salt and pepper.

3. Stir together the shredded coconut and hazelnut in a small bowl.

4. Dredge the fish fillets in the coconut mixture so that both sides of each piece are thickly coated.

5. Put the fish on the baking sheet and lightly brush both sides of each piece with the coconut oil.

6. Bake the haddock until the topping is golden and the fish flakes easily with a fork, about 12 minutes total. Serve.

Nutrition:

Calories 299

Fat 24g

Protein 20g

Carbs 1g

38.   Simple Keto Fried Chicken

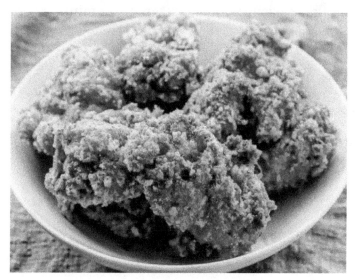

Preparation time: 15 minutes

Cooking time: 45 minutes

Servings: 4

Ingredients:

- 4 boneless chicken thighs

- Frying oil

- 2 eggs

- 2tablespoon. heavy whipping cream

- Breading

- 2/3cup grated parmesan cheese

- 2/3cup blanched almond flour

- 1teaspoon. salt

- ½teaspoon. black pepper

- ½teaspoon. cayenne

- ½teaspoon. paprika

Directions:

1. Beat the eggs and heavy cream. Separately, mix all the breading fixing. Set aside.

2. Cut the chicken thigh into 3 even pieces.

3. Dip the chicken in the bread first before dipping it in the egg wash and then finally, dipping it in the breading again. Fry chicken within 5 minutes. Pat dry the chicken. Serve.

Nutrition:

Calories: 304

Carbs: 12g

Fat: 15g

Protein: 30g

39. Keto Butter Chicken

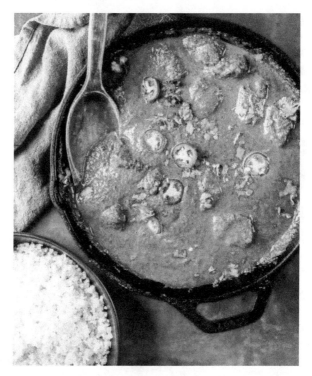

Preparation time: 15 minutes

Cooking time: 20 minutes

Servings: 4

Ingredients:

- 1.5lb. chicken breast

- 1tablespoon. coconut oil

- 2tablespoon. garam masala

- 3teaspoon. grated ginger

- 3teaspoon. garlic

- 4oz. plain yogurt

- Sauce:

- 2tablespoon. butter

- 1tablespoon ground coriander

- ½cup heavy cream

- ½tablespoon. garam masala

- 2teaspoon. ginger

- 2teaspoon. minced garlic

- 2teaspoon. cumin

- 1teaspoon. chili powder

- 1 onion

- 14.5oz. crushed tomatoes

- Salt

Directions:

1. Mix chicken pieces, 2 tablespoons garam masala, 1 teaspoon minced garlic, and 1 teaspoon grated ginger. Stir and add the yogurt. Chill for 30 minutes.

2. For the sauce, blend the ginger, garlic, onion, tomatoes, and spices. Put aside.

3. Cook the chicken pieces. Once cooked, pour in the sauce, and simmer for 5 minutes. Serve.

Nutrition:

Calories: 367

Carbs: 7g

Fat: 22g

Protein: 36g

40. Keto Shrimp Scampi Recipe

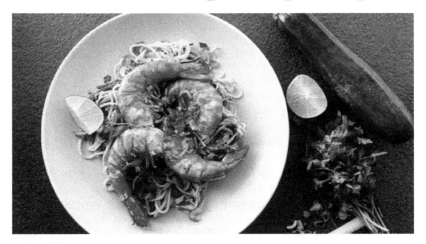

Preparation time: 15 minutes

Cooking time: 25 minutes

Servings: 2

Ingredients:

- 2 summer squash

- 1-pound shrimp

- 2tablespoon. butter unsalted

- 2tablespoon. lemon juice

- 2tablespoon. parsley

- ¼cup chicken broth

- 1/8teaspoon. red chili flakes

- 1 clove garlic

- Salt

- pepper

Directions:

1. Put salt in the squash noodles on top. Set aside for 30 minutes.

2. Pat dry. Fry the garlic. Add some chicken broth, red chili flakes, and lemon juice.

3. Once it boils, add the shrimp, and cook. Lower the heat.

4. Add salt and pepper, put the summer squash noodles and parsley to the mix. Serve.

Nutrition:

Calories: 366

Carbs: 7g

Fat: 15g

Protein: 49g

Vegetarians

41.   Berries & Spinach Salad

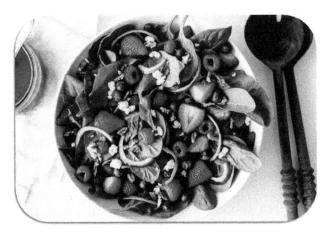

Preparation time: 10 minutes

Cooking time: 0 minutes

Servings: 5

Ingredients:

Salad

- 8 cups fresh baby spinach
- ¾ cup fresh strawberries, hulled and sliced
- ¾ cup fresh blueberries
- ¼ cup onion, sliced
- ¼ cup almond, sliced
- ¼ cup feta cheese, crumbled

Dressing

- 1/3 cup olive oil

- 2 tablespoons fresh lemon juice

- ¼ teaspoon liquid stevia

- 1/8 teaspoon garlic powder

- Salt, to taste

Directions:

1. For salad: In a bowl, add the spinach, berries, onion, and almonds, and mix.

2. For dressing: In another small bowl, add all the ingredients and beat until well combined.

3. Place the dressing over salad and gently, toss to coat well.

Nutrition:

Calories 190

Net Carbs 6 g

Total Fat 17.2 g

Saturated Fat 3.3 g

Cholesterol 7 mg

Sodium 145 mg

Total Carbs 8.5 g

Fiber 2.5 g

Sugar 4.6 g - Protein 3.3 g

42. Egg & Avocado Salad

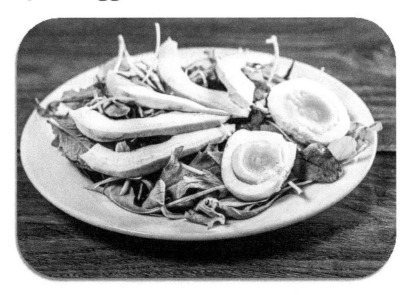

Preparation time: 10 minutes

Cooking time: 0 minutes

Servings: 4

Ingredients:

Dressing

- 3 tablespoons olive oil

- 1 tablespoon fresh lime juice

- Salt and ground black pepper, to taste

Salad

- 5 cups fresh baby greens

- 4 hard-boiled organic eggs, peeled and sliced

- 2 avocados; peeled, pitted, and sliced

- 2 tablespoons fresh mint leaves

Directions:

4. For dressing: Place oil, lime juice, salt, and black pepper in a small bowl and beat until well combined.

5. Divide the spinach onto serving plates and top each with tuna, egg, cucumber, and tomato.

6. Drizzle with dressing and serve.

Nutrition:

Calories 332

Net Carbs 2.5 g

Total Fat 31.5 g

Saturated Fat 6.4 g

Cholesterol 164 mg

Sodium 111 mg

Total Carbs 8.8 g

Fiber 6.3 g

Sugar 1.2 g

Protein 7.7 g

43.   Tomato, Arugula & Mozzarella Salad

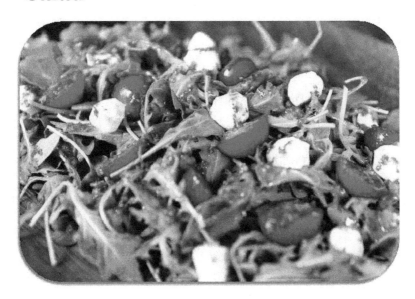

Preparation time: 15 minutes

Cooking time: 0 minutes

Servings: 4

Ingredients:

Dressing

- ½ cup fresh basil leaves

- 2 garlic cloves, peeled

- 4 tablespoons olive oil

- 2 tablespoon balsamic vinegar

- Salt and ground black pepper, to taste

Salad

- 2 cups cherry tomatoes

- 3 ounces mozzarella cheese balls

- 5 cups fresh arugula

Directions:

1. For filling: In a small blender, add all the ingredients and pulse until smooth.

2. For salad: In a large bowl, add all the ingredients and mix.

3. Place the dressing over salad and toss to coat well.

4. Serve immediately.

Nutrition:

Calories 207

Net Carbs 4.2 g

Total Fat 18.1 g

Saturated Fat 4.3 g

Cholesterol 11 mg

Sodium 178 mg

Total Carbs 5.8 g

Fiber 1.6 g

Sugar 2.9 g

Protein 7.6 g

44. Smoked Salmon & Zucchini Salad

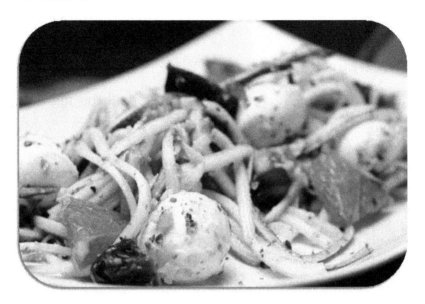

Preparation time: 10 minutes

Cooking time: 0 minutes

Servings: 4

Ingredients:

Dressing

- 3 tablespoons olive oil

- 2 tablespoons balsamic vinegar

- ½ tablespoon Dijon mustard

- ¼ teaspoon red pepper flakes, crushed

Salad

- 12 ounces smoked salmon

- 3 medium zucchinis, spiralized with blade C

- 1 cup fresh mozzarella balls

- 2 tablespoons fresh basil, chopped

Directions:

1. For dressing: In a small blender, add all the ingredients and pulse until smooth.

2. For salad: In a large bowl, add all the ingredients and mix.

3. Place the dressing over salad and toss to coat well.

4. Serve immediately.

Nutrition:

Calories 158

Net Carbs 2.4 g

Total Fat 10.5 g

Saturated Fat 2.1 g

Cholesterol 16 mg

Sodium 1,100 mg

Total Carbs 3.6 g

Fiber 1.2 g

Sugar 1.7 g

Protein 13 g

45. Cucumber & Tomato Salad

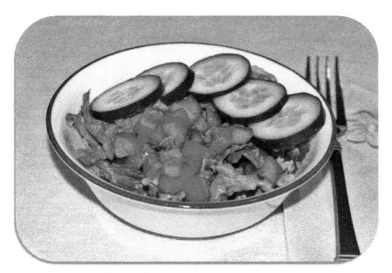

Preparation time: 15 minutes

Cooking time: 0 minutes

Servings: 4

Ingredients:

- Salad

- 3 large English cucumbers, thinly sliced

- 2 cups tomatoes, chopped

- 6 cups lettuce, torn

- Dressing

- 4 tablespoons olive oil

- 2 tablespoons balsamic vinegar

- 1 tablespoon fresh lemon juice

- Salt and ground black pepper, as required

Directions:

1. For salad: In a large bowl, add the cucumbers, onion, cucumbers, and mix.

2. For dressing: In a small bowl, add all the ingredients and beat until well combined.

3. Place the dressing over the salad and toss to coat well.

4. Serve immediately.

Nutrition:

Calories 86

Net Carbs 0 g

Total Fat 7.3 g

Saturated Fat 1 g

Cholesterol 0 mg

Sodium 27 mg

Total Carbs 5.1 g

Fiber 1.4 g

Sugar 2.8 g

Protein 1.1 g

46.   Creamy Shrimp Salad

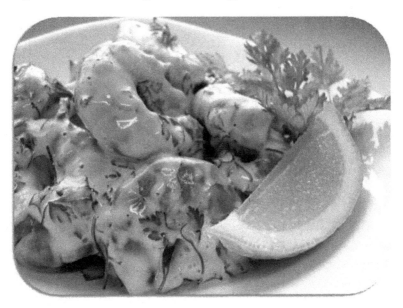

Preparation time: 15 minutes

Cooking time: 0 minutes

Servings: 4

Ingredients:

- ¼ cup sour cream

- 2 tablespoons mayonnaise

- 2 tablespoons fresh lemon juice

- 1 teaspoon Old Bay seasoning

- Salt, to taste

- 16 ounces cooked shrimp

- 2 medium cucumbers, peeled and chopped

- 3 tablespoons fresh parsley, chopped

Directions:

1. Add sour cream, mayonnaise, lime juice, Old Bay, and salt in a large salad bowl and mix well.

2. Add remaining ingredients and gently, stir to combine.

3. Refrigerate to chill before serving.

Nutrition:

Calories 225

Net Carbs 4.9 g

Total Fat 10.1 g

Saturated Fat 3.3 g

Cholesterol 248 mg

Sodium 533 mg

Total Carbs 5.4 g

Fiber 0.5 g

Sugar 1.5 g

Protein 26.9 g

47. Salmon Salad

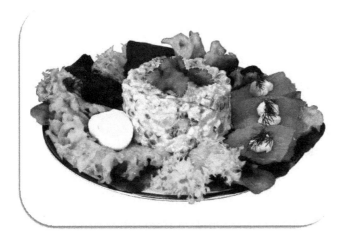

Preparation time: 20 minutes

Cooking time: 0 minutes

Servings: 4

Ingredients:

- 12 hard-boiled organic eggs, peeled and cubed

- 1 pound smoked salmon

- 3 celery stalks, chopped

- 1 yellow onion, chopped

- 4 tablespoons fresh dill, chopped

- 2 cups mayonnaise

- Salt and ground black pepper, as required

- 8 cups fresh lettuce leaves

Directions:

1. In a large serving bowl, add all the ingredients (except the lettuce leaves) and gently stir to combine.

2. Cover and refrigerate to chill before serving.

3. Divide the lettuce onto serving plates and top with the salmon salad.

4. Serve immediately.

Nutrition:

Calories 539

Net Carbs 3.5 g

Total Fat 49.2 g

Saturated Fat 8.6 g

Cholesterol 279 mg

Sodium 1618 mg

Total Carbs 4.5 g

Fiber 1 g

Sugar 1.7 g

Protein 19.4 g

48. Chicken & Strawberry Salad

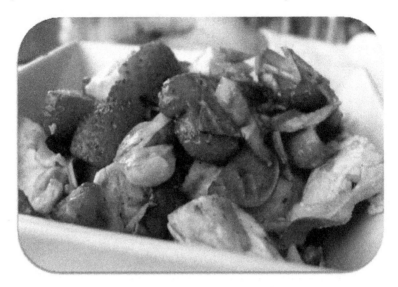

Preparation time: 15 minutes

Cooking time: 0 minutes

Servings: 4

Ingredients:

- 2 pounds grass-fed boneless skinless chicken breasts

- ½ cup olive oil

- ¼ cup fresh lemon juice

- 2 tablespoons granulated erythritol

- 1 garlic clove, minced

- Salt and ground black pepper, as required

- 4 cups fresh strawberries

- 8 cups fresh spinach, torn

Directions:

1. For marinade: in a large bowl, add oil, lemon juice, erythritol, garlic, salt, and black pepper, and beat until well combined.

2. In a large resealable plastic bag, place the chicken and ¾ cup of marinade.

3. Seal bag and shake to coat well.

4. Refrigerate overnight.

5. Cover the bowl of remaining marinade and refrigerate before serving.

6. Preheat the grill to medium heat. Grease the grill grate.

7. Remove the chicken from bag and discard the marinade.

8. Place the chicken onto grill grate and grill, covered for about 5–8 minutes per side.

9. Remove chicken from grill and cut into bite sized pieces.

10. In a large bowl, add the chicken pieces, strawberries, and spinach, and mix.

11. Place the reserved marinade and toss to coat.

12. Serve immediately.

Nutrition:

Calories 356

Net Carbs 4 g

Total Fat 21.4 g

Saturated Fat 4 g

Cholesterol 101 mg

Sodium 143 mg

Total Carbs 6.1 g

Fiber 2.1 g

Sugar 3.8 g

Protein 34.2 g

49.   tomato & mozzarella salad

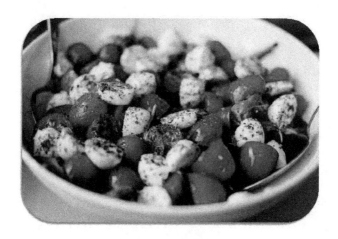

Preparation time: 10 minutes

Cooking time: 0 minutes

Servings: 4

Ingredients:

- 4 cups cherry tomatoes, halved
- 1½ pounds mozzarella cheese, cubed
- ¼ cup fresh basil leaves, chopped
- ¼ cup olive oil
- 2 tablespoons fresh lemon juice
- 1 teaspoon fresh oregano, minced
- 1 teaspoon fresh parsley, minced
- 2–4 drops liquid stevia

- Salt and ground black pepper, as required

Directions:

1. In a salad bowl, mix together tomatoes, mozzarella, and basil.

2. In a small bowl, add remaining ingredients and beat until well combined.

3. Place dressing over salad and toss to coat well.

4. Serve immediately.

Nutrition:

Calories 87

Net Carbs 2.7 g

Total Fat 7.5 g

Saturated Fat 1.5 g

Cholesterol 3 mg

Sodium 57 mg

Total Carbs 3.9 g

Fiber 1.2 g

Sugar 2.5 g

Protein 2.4 g

50. Shrimp Salad

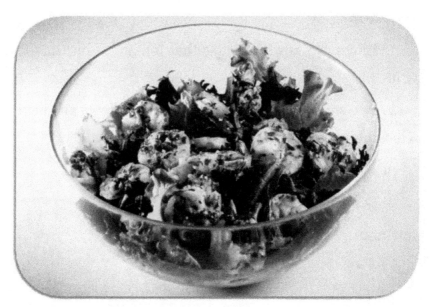

Preparation time: 15 minutes

Cooking time: 15 minutes

Servings: 6

Ingredients:

- 1 tablespoon unsalted butter

- 1 garlic clove, crushed and divided

- 2 tablespoons fresh rosemary, chopped

- 1 pound shrimp, peeled and deveined

- Salt and ground black pepper, as required

- 4 cups fresh arugula

- 2 cups lettuce, torn

- 2 tablespoons olive oil

- 2 tablespoons fresh lime juice

Directions:

1. In a large wok, melt the butter over medium heat and sauté 1 garlic clove for about 1 minute.

2. Add the shrimp with salt and black pepper and cook for about 4–5 minutes.

3. Remove from the heat and set aside to cool.

4. Ina large bowl, add the shrimp, arugula, oil, lime juice, salt, and black pepper, and gently toss to coat.

5. Serve immediately.

Nutrition:

Calories 157

Net Carbs 2.3 g

Total Fat 8.2 g

Saturated Fat 2.4 g

Cholesterol 164 mg

Sodium 230 mg

Total Carbs 3.1 g

Fiber 0.8 g

Sugar 0.5 g

Protein 17.7 g

CPSIA information can be obtained
at www.ICGtesting.com
Printed in the USA
LVHW080810220221
679596LV00025B/1268

9 781801 767644